JUICING FOR CANCER

Nourish Your Body, Fight Back and Thrive

Dr. Rachel Ferguson

.

TABLE OF CONTENTS

INTRODUCTION 5

Cancer-fighting fruits and vegetables 8

Cruciferous Vegetables: 8

Berries: 9

Leafy Greens: 10

Recipes for Cancer-Fighting Juices 11

Green Juice Recipe: 11

Berry Blast Juice Recipe: 12

Citrus Sunrise Juice Recipe: 13

Breakfast Recipes 15

Green Breakfast Juice: 15

Berry Oatmeal Smoothie: 16

Lunch Recipes 17

Immunity-Boosting Juice:......................17

Green Vegetable Juice:..........................18

Dinner Recipes 19

Antioxidant-Rich Veggie Juice:...........19

Carrot-Ginger Detox Juice: 20

Conclusion and Final Tips 22

Contact Us:

You can also contact us in our 24hrs email address for guidance or advice. **mailto:drrachelferguson@gmail.com**

Reach out below to see more of our health books and lots more in our store!

Drrachelferguson

Appreciation

We would be forever grateful if you could take a few moments after you've finished reading, to leave us a positive review on Amazon. Your review will not only help us to reach a wider audience, but it will also help other readers to discover the value of our book. We know that your time is valuable, so we truly appreciate your willingness to share your thoughts with us. Thank you in advance for your kind review.

INTRODUCTION

Juicing has gained popularity as a dietary approach offering potential cancer patient benefits. While it is important to note that juicing alone is not a cure for cancer, it can be a complementary strategy to support overall health and wellbeing during cancer treatment. Here are some potential benefits of juicing for cancer patients:

Increased Nutrient Intake: Juicing allows cancer patients to consume a concentrated amount of nutrients from fruits and vegetables in an easily digestible form. Freshly extracted juices provide vitamins, minerals, antioxidants, and phytochemicals that are essential for optimal health and can support the body's natural defenses.

Hydration Support: Staying hydrated is crucial for cancer patients, especially those undergoing treatments like chemotherapy that can cause dehydration. Juices are a hydrating option that can contribute to maintaining proper fluid balance in the body.

Antioxidant and Anti-inflammatory Support: Many fruits and vegetables used in juicing are rich in antioxidants, which help neutralize harmful free radicals and reduce oxidative stress. Chronic inflammation is often associated with cancer, and specific ingredients used in juicing, such as turmeric and ginger, possess anti-inflammatory properties.

Promoting Detoxification: Juicing can support the body's natural detoxification processes by providing nutrients that aid liver function. Ingredients like leafy greens, beets, and citrus fruits are known for their detoxifying properties, assisting in eliminating toxins from the body.

Digestive Health Support: Cancer treatments and medications can sometimes affect the digestive system, leading to challenges such as poor appetite, nausea, or difficulty absorbing nutrients. Juicing offers a way to obtain essential nutrients while reducing the digestive burden, as fiber is removed during juicing.

Alleviating Nutritional Challenges: Cancer patients often face nutritional challenges due to appetite changes, taste alterations, or difficulty swallowing.

Juicing can be a convenient way to consume various fruits and vegetables, providing a nutrient-dense option that is easier to consume and digest.

Cancer patients must consult their healthcare professionals before incorporating juicing into their treatment plans. They can guide specific dietary considerations based on the patient's needs, treatment protocols, and any potential interactions with medications. Juicing should be seen as a complementary strategy alongside a well-balanced diet, not as a replacement for medical advice and treatments.

Cancer-fighting fruits and vegetables

Incorporating cancer-fighting fruits and vegetables into your recipes can provide additional nutritional benefits when it comes to juicing for cancer. Here are some examples of fruits and vegetables known for their potential cancer-fighting properties:

Cruciferous Vegetables:

Broccoli: Contains sulforaphane, which has shown anticancer properties and supports detoxification enzymes.

Kale: Packed with antioxidants, vitamins, and minerals that may help protect against certain cancers.

Cabbage: Rich in glucosinolates, converted into compounds that may inhibit cancer cell growth.

Berries:

Blueberries: Loaded with antioxidants, including anthocyanins, which have been linked to reduced cancer risk.

Strawberries: Contain ellagic acid and vitamin C, known for their potential anticancer effects.

Raspberries: High in ellagic acid and other phytochemicals that may help inhibit tumor growth.

Citrus Fruits:

Oranges: Rich in vitamin C and other antioxidants that support immune function and protect against oxidative damage.

Lemons: Packed with vitamin C and limonoids, which may have anticancer properties?

Grapefruits: Contain the antioxidant compound lycopene and other phytochemicals associated with reduced cancer risk.

Leafy Greens:

Spinach: Provides foliate, antioxidants, and chlorophyll, which may help protect against various cancers.

Swiss Chard: Rich in vitamins A, C, and K, as well as fiber and phytochemicals that promote overall health.

Kale contains abundant antioxidants, fiber, and other compounds with potential anticancer properties.

Turmeric and Ginger:

Turmeric contains curcumin, a potent anti-inflammatory, and antioxidant compound that may help inhibit cancer cell growth.

Ginger: Known for its anti-inflammatory properties and potential to reduce the risk of certain cancers.

Recipes for Cancer-Fighting Juices

Green Juice Recipe:

Ingredients:

- 2 cups spinach
- 1 cucumber
- 2 celery stalks
- 1 green apple
- ½ lemons (peeled)
- 1-inch piece of ginger

Instructions:

Wash all the ingredients thoroughly.

Chop the cucumber, celery, and green apple into small pieces.

Add all the ingredients to a juicer.

Process them until well blended and smooth.

Pour the juice into a glass and consume immediately.

Berry Blast Juice Recipe:

Ingredients:

- 1 cup strawberries
- 1 cup blueberries
- ½ cup raspberries
- 1 small beet (peeled and chopped)
- 1 carrot (peeled and chopped)
- 1 cup coconut water

Instructions:

Rinse the berries and remove any stems.

Add the strawberries, blueberries, raspberries, beet, and carrots to a juicer.

Juice the ingredients until well combined.

Stir in the coconut water.

Transfer the juice to a glass and enjoy.

Citrus Sunrise Juice Recipe:

Ingredients:

- 2 oranges (peeled)
- 1 grapefruit (peeled)
- 3 carrots (peeled and chopped)
- 1-inch piece of turmeric root (or 1 teaspoon of ground turmeric)

Instructions:

Wash and chop the oranges, grapefruit, and carrots.

Add all the ingredients to a juicer.

Juice the ingredients until well blended.

Pour the juice into a glass.

If using ground turmeric, sprinkle it on top and stir well.

Drink the juice immediately.

Use fresh and organic produce whenever possible to maximize the nutritional benefits. Feel free to adjust the ingredient quantities based on your taste preferences. It's essential to consult with your healthcare professional before incorporating these recipes into your diet, especially if you are currently undergoing cancer treatment. They can provide personalized advice and guidance based on your health condition and treatment plan.

Breakfast Recipes

Green Breakfast Juice:

Ingredients:

- 2 cups spinach
- 1 cucumber
- 2 celery stalks
- 1 green apple
- ½ Lemon (peeled)
- 1-inch piece of ginger

Instructions:

Wash all the ingredients thoroughly.

Chop the cucumber, celery, and green apple into small pieces.

Add all the ingredients to a juicer.

Process them until well blended and smooth.

Pour the juice into a glass and enjoy it as a refreshing and nutritious breakfast option.

Berry Oatmeal Smoothie:

Ingredients:

- 1 cup mixed berries (e.g., blueberries, strawberries, raspberries)
- ½ cup rolled oats
- 1 ripe banana
- 1 cup almond milk (or any preferred plant-based milk)
- 1 tablespoon chia seeds
- 1 tablespoon honey (optional)

Instructions:

Rinse the berries and remove any stems.

Add all the ingredients to a blender.

Blend on high until smooth and creamy.

If desired, add honey for additional sweetness.

Pour the smoothie into a glass and enjoy it alongside your breakfast or as a standalone meal.

Lunch Recipes

Immunity-Boosting Juice:

Ingredients:

- 2 carrots (peeled and chopped)
- 1 small beet (peeled and chopped)
- 1 inch of fresh turmeric root (or 1 teaspoon of ground turmeric)
- 1 inch of fresh ginger root
- 1 orange (peeled)
- ½ Lemon (peeled)
- 1 cup coconut water

Instructions:

Wash and prepare all the ingredients.

Add the carrots, beet, turmeric, ginger, orange, and lemon to a juicer.

Juice the ingredients until well blended.

Stir in the coconut water.

Pour the juice into a glass and enjoy it as a nutrient-packed lunch option.

Green Vegetable Juice:

Ingredients:

- 2 cups spinach
- 1 cucumber
- 2 stalks of celery
- ½ Green bell pepper
- ½ Lemon (peeled)
- Handful of fresh parsley

Instructions:

Wash all the ingredients thoroughly.

Chop the cucumber, celery, and green bell pepper into small pieces.

Add all the ingredients to a juicer.

Process them until well blended and smooth.

Pour the juice into a glass and enjoy it as a refreshing and nutritious lunch option.

Dinner Recipes

Antioxidant-Rich Veggie Juice:

Ingredients:

- 2 large tomatoes

- 2 carrots (peeled and chopped)

- 1 red bell pepper

- 2 stalks of celery

- ½ beet (peeled and chopped)

- Handful of fresh basil leaves

Instructions:

Wash and prepare all the ingredients.

Cut the tomatoes and red bell pepper into chunks.

Add all the ingredients to a juicer.

Process them until well blended and smooth.

Pour the juice into a glass and enjoy it as a refreshing and nutritious dinner option.

Carrot-Ginger Detox Juice:

Ingredients:

- 4 large carrots (peeled and chopped)
- 1 inch of fresh ginger root
- 1 small apple
- ½ Lemon (peeled)
- Handful of fresh mint leaves

Instructions:

Wash and prepare all the ingredients.

Chop the carrots and apples into small pieces.

Add all the ingredients to a juicer.

Process them until well blended and smooth.

Pour the juice into a glass and enjoy it as a cleansing and nutritious dinner option.

These recipes incorporate cancer-fighting ingredients like tomatoes, carrots, bell peppers, ginger, and lemon. Adjust the ingredient quantities based on your taste preferences.

Remember to consult your healthcare professional before making significant dietary changes, especially when undergoing cancer treatment. They can provide personalized advice based on your health condition and treatment plan.

Conclusion and Final Tips

Incorporating juicing into a cancer-fighting diet can provide a convenient and nutritious way to support your overall health and wellbeing. While juicing alone is not a cure for cancer, it can complement your treatment plan by providing a concentrated dose of essential nutrients, antioxidants, and phytochemicals.

Here are some final tips to keep in mind:

Please consult with a Healthcare Professional: Before making any significant changes to your diet, it is essential to consult with your healthcare professional or a registered dietitian who specializes in oncology. They can provide personalized advice based on your health condition, treatment plan, and dietary needs.

Choose Fresh and Organic Produce: Opt for fresh, organic fruits and vegetables whenever possible to ensure maximum nutrient content and minimize exposure to harmful chemicals.

Variety is Key: Incorporate a variety of fruits, vegetables, and herbs in your juicing recipes to obtain a broad spectrum of nutrients and phytochemicals.

Balance Your Ingredients: Aim for a balance of leafy greens, cruciferous vegetables, berries, citrus fruits, and anti-inflammatory ingredients like turmeric and ginger to maximize the cancer-fighting potential of your juices.

Drink Immediately: Freshly juiced fruits and vegetables are most nutritious when consumed immediately. Avoid storing juices for extended periods as they may lose some nutritional value.

Consider Fiber Intake: Juicing removes the fiber from fruits and vegetables. While this can make nutrients more easily absorbed, consuming whole fruits, vegetables, and other high-fiber foods is essential to support digestion and overall gut health.

Personalize and Enjoy: Adjust the recipes to your taste preferences and experiment with different combinations of ingredients. Make juicing a part of a balanced and varied diet, and don't forget to savor and enjoy the flavors!